1-2-3

1-2-3

The Three Steps THAT CREATE Weight Success

John D. Correll

Fulfillment Press
U.S.A.

Title: 1-2-3

Subtitle: The Three Steps THAT CREATE Weight Success

Fulfillment Press | U.S.A.

ISBN: 978-1-938001-96-3
Amazon URL: amazon.com/dp/1938001966
Version: TXT 2024-1-1 (8) | COV 2024-1-1 (3)

Fulfillment Press is an imprint and a dba of Correll Consulting, LLC.

John Correll enjoys walking, biking, sight-seeing with his family, creating photographs, book publishing, and reading American history and positive psychology. More on him can be found at: correllconcepts.com/correll_bio.htm
(Note: This is not the same John Correll who creates the excellent children's books.)

Disclaimer: Before beginning any diet or weight management program, or making a major change to a present dietary program, a licensed physician should be consulted. If any information in this book should contradict or conflict with any prescription or advice of your physician or chosen dietary program, we recommend you ignore and do not apply whatever that conflicting information contained in this book might be. This book is not a dietary guide.

For additional resources and books by John Correll, go to: http://correllconcepts.com

KINDLE VERSION – If, in addition to this paper book, you would like to have a handy Kindle version too — which can be accessed and read on your computer, tablet, and/or smartphone — go to: Amazon.com/dp/B0CQGGWNMM

I dedicate this book to you, the Reader. May you live out your life in your desired weight range and strive to become the finest person you're capable of being and help others to do the same.

Special thanks to my wife and life partner Janet for triggering my initial search beginning in 2006 for the cause of why a few persons are succeeding at creating healthy-weight living while most are not.

CONTENTS

INTRODUCTION

Research studies tell us that about ninety percent of persons who lose a substantial amount of weight eventually have it all come back BUT ten percent keep the lost weight off forever. This book tells you **WHY** that situation is happening and **HOW** you can be one of the ten percent who succeed at living their desired weight forever.

The first thing to know is:

This is <u>not</u> a weight *control* book.

It's a weight *success* book.

Weight Success is: Living most or all of your days in your desired healthy-weight range <u>and</u> deriving benefit from it.

Creating weight success involves *three* steps — which I've dubbed Step 1, Step 2, Step 3. But before describing them I must explain two concepts.

CONCEPT 1:
Two Types of Persons

Regarding weight success there are two types of persons. I call them Type 1 and Type 2.

Type 1 are those who automatically experience weight success throughout their life. Meaning, they get it without taking any deliberate actions to create it. It just sort of "magically happens" for them.

Type 2 are those who experience weight success only by performing certain steps to make it happen. When they apply these certain steps they succeed at living in their desired weight range. When they don't apply these steps they *don't* succeed at living in their desired weight range.

You also need to know that some Type 2 persons appear to be Type 1 when they're young. But, actually they're a "late blooming" Type 2. This becomes apparent when they reach early or middle adulthood and start gaining weight.

Now here's a key point. Only a small percentage of persons are **Type 1** — I suspect it's around 10 percent.

Everyone else, including me, is **Type 2.**
Type 2's make up the big majority of the
population. The rest of this book is intended
for Type 2's. So, from hereon when I speak
of "persons" or "people" I'm referring to
Type 2 persons.

CONCEPT 2:
Weight Success Boils Down to Doing Three Basic Steps

After sixteen years of observing, experiment-
ing, reading, applying, and writing about
weight control I discovered something big.
It turned out to be the diamond in the
weight-information dung heap. I discovered
that weight success is created by doing
three basic actions.

I call these three basic actions the *3-step
Process to Weight Success.*

By doing this 3-step Process a human succeeds at creating weight success.

By <u>not</u> doing this Process a person likely *doesn't* succeed at creating weight success. Now here are the three Steps of the Process.

Step 1: Decide that you're going to live the rest of your life in your desired healthy-weight range.

Step 2: Select, or create, an action plan — such as, for example, a certain dietary (or eating) plan — that you believe will be most effective in creating weight success for *you.*

Step 3: Do the action plan in *entirety.*

Doing the plan in entirety means, if the plan has a prescribed set of daily weight-success-creating actions that you're supposed to do each day, then do those actions <u>each</u> day (or at least most days).

So, to sum up:

Step 1 is the DECISION step.

Step 2 is the ACTION PLAN SELECTION step.

Step 3 is the DAILY DO-IT step.

That's the **1-2-3** of creating lifelong weight success.

I realize all this might appear overly simplistic. But keep this in mind. Doing the 3-step Process to Weight Success is how overeating and weight gain are conquered.

It's also how successful weight reduction happens.

And, it's also how lost weight is kept off.

In short, for the vast majority of persons, it's the process by which ongoing weight success is realized.

That is the epiphany that finally came to me after sixteen years of formulating, refining, testing, and personally creating ongoing weight success.

Moving on, it's important to know that each action in this 3-step Process is critical.

If you don't do Step 1 the process never gets started.

If you do Step 1 but not Step 2, the process likely will abort at that point.

And, if you do Steps 1 and 2 but not Step 3, you eventually will quit pursuing weight control due to repeated failure and frustration. So, all three steps are vital for creating weight success.

You now know what you need to do to succeed at creating lifelong weight success. So at this point, if you prefer, you can stop reading and begin applying the 3-step Process to Weight Success. And remember, the first step is: Decide that you're going to live the rest of your life in your desired healthy-weight range.

BUT, in case you first might like a little more information on this Process, I'll continue explaining. Here in greater detail are the three steps to weight success.

STEP 1:
The Decision Step

In this step you decide that you're going to live the rest of your life in your desired healthy-weight range.

As already stated, *weight success* is the situation in which you're living most or all of your days in your desired healthy-weight range <u>and</u> deriving benefit from it.

A few rare persons stumble upon weight success by accident.

But for the majority of us, succeeding at creating weight success begins with a certain *decision.* It's the decision to cease living overweight and to begin living in our desired weight range.

I call this the *weight success decision.* Making this decision is the crucial first step to succeeding at achieving weight success. The more firm and resolute this decision is, the better for you.

So, I suggest you decide that living at your desired weight range is a mandatory feature of your life. *Mandatory feature* means: <u>non</u>-optional, <u>will</u>-do, <u>must</u>-have aspect of your existence.

Also, keep this in mind. Most persons who fail to create weight success have also failed to make the decision that living in their desired weight range is a *mandatory* feature of their life.

Here's why that happens. When living in your desired weight range *isn't* a mandatory, must-have aspect of your life, you tend to get discouraged or quit whenever the first little setback or challenge arises.

So, decide right now that living in your desired weight range is — and will continue to be — a *mandatory* feature of your exist-ence. Then, hold this decision in mind every day.

STEP 2:
The Action Plan Selection Step

In this step you select, or create, an action plan — such as, for example, a certain eating (or dietary or weight success) plan — that you believe will be most effective in creating weight success for YOU.

To begin I must lay down three facts.

First, no weight success action plan —
a.k.a. dietary or eating program — is "a best
action plan for everyone." Meaning, the best
or most effective action plan for me might
not be the best action plan for you.

Second, the best action plan for each of
us is the plan by which we can get the best
results. And, perhaps also the easiest
results.

Third, the degree of best results that you
derive from any action plan is affected by
your mindset — or the beliefs and feelings
you hold about the plan. This is because
productive beliefs and feelings create
productive actions and results (and counterproductive beliefs and feelings create
counterproductive actions and results).

So, your goal should be to find, or create,
the most effective action plan for YOU. Here
are four thoughts on how you might do that.

FIRST, do some research on major weight control programs presently on the market. So, which programs are the "major" ones? I suggest you assume that any weight success program that's doing TV advertising qualifies as a "major weight success program."

Also, assume that any program that has a book or major literature about it is a "major" program.

> **Note:** I am not saying that being "major" automatically means it's "good" or "most effective."

Finally, do some online research. Check out websites, post questions on search engines, and/or inquire on social media.

SECOND, talk with anyone you know who is now, or has been, doing a particular weight success program. Find out how it worked for them, what they liked and disliked.

THIRD, if it turns out that none of the present weight success programs appear to be perfect for you, then you might consider creating your own weight success program.

> **Note:** If you go down the create-it-yourself road, make *certain* that the program — a.k.a. action plan — that you create comprises only healthy eating practices and no harmful actions.

FOURTH, if none of the above suggestions reveals a best-possible weight success program, or action plan, for you, then consider devising a *hybrid* weight success program. That is, combine two programs that are presently available. Take a portion of one program and combine it with a portion of another program.

> **Final Note:** If it happens you'd like to check out the action plan used by the author of this book, get the book titled *The Key to Weight Success* and then read Chapter **3**. It describes an action plan known as the Weight Success Method.

STEP 3:
The Daily Do-it Step

In this step you do the action plan in entirety.

Which means:

If the plan calls for doing certain *start-up* actions, DO those start-up actions.

If the plan calls for doing certain *daily* actions, DO those daily actions every day (or at least most days).

If the plan calls for doing certain *periodic* actions, DO those periodic actions when they're supposed to be done.

This Step 3 is where the rubber meets the road. Doing Steps 1 and 2 are pointless if you don't do this one thing: Do your selected dietary, eating, or weight success action plan *fully.*

So, you now come to a pivotal decision. I call it the "Next-step Decision." Here's an infographic of it:

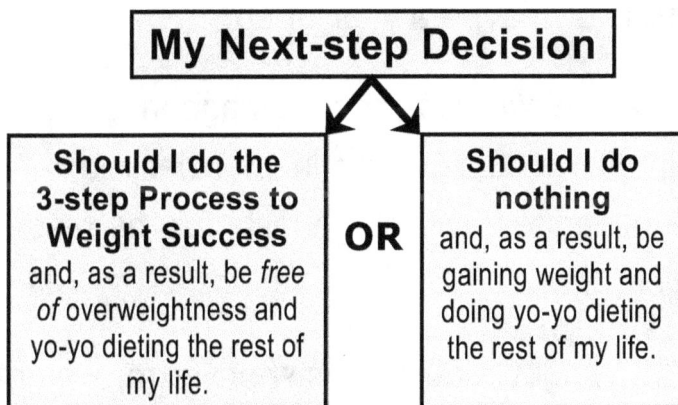

My Next-step Decision	
Should I do the 3-step Process to Weight Success and, as a result, be *free of* overweightness and yo-yo dieting the rest of my life.	**OR** **Should I do nothing** and, as a result, be gaining weight and doing yo-yo dieting the rest of my life.

Now, here's a vital thing you need to know. Lifelong weight success is a two-stage process. Here's how it works.

THE TWO STAGES OF WEIGHT SUCCESS

For most persons weight success comes in two stages: (1) weight reduction stage and (2) weight maintenance stage.

The *weight reduction* stage involves losing weight until you reach your desired weight. This stage lasts for perhaps a few months or maybe a year or so.

The *weight maintenance* stage involves maintaining your weight in your desired weight range. This stage lasts for the rest of your life.

So, weight reduction is short term; weight maintenance is forever. Now here's a key point.

One of the biggest factors that cause many persons to fail at creating lifelong weight success is this. They assume that creating weight success is a 1-stage game — that it's only about succeeding at weight reduction.

But, there's a problem with viewing weight success as a 1-stage game. Once a person reaches their desired weight it causes them to conclude "the weight game is won."

So, then what happens? First, the person celebrates, or at least feels good about, their weight reduction accomplishment. (And they *should* feel good about it because it's a substantial accomplishment.)

Then, they do *nothing* — that is, they do nothing significant pertaining to creating weight maintenance.

What's the inevitable heart-breaking outcome? *They gradually gain back all the weight they lost.*

In short, weight maintenance does not derive from "doing nothing." To create weight maintenance a person must "do something." And, specifically, what they must do is this: Continue doing Step 3 (the Daily Do-it step) for the rest of their life.

So, to sum up, creating lifelong weight success involves two stages. First, a short-term stage of weight reduction. Followed by a lifelong stage of weight maintenance. And the key to success in each of the stages is: Doing the 3-step Process to Weight Success.

> **NOTE:** Even though the 3-step Process is used for both stages it doesn't mean the action plan (step 2) is the same for both stages. The weight maintenance stage might require a slightly different action plan than what's used in the weight reduction stage.

Now I'm going to take a short side-ride to give you one of the most mind-blowing insights of the "weight control world."

THE WEIGHT REGAIN PROBLEM ... AND THE FIX

For decades now weight loss research data have disclosed a scary phenomenon.

It tells us that about 90 percent of the times when people lose a large amount of weight they gain it back. It might happen quickly or maybe over a longer time like a year or two. But eventually, in about nine out of ten instances a person gains back all the weight they lost — and usually more.

So, this sad situation forces a key question:

*WHY is it that about **90** percent of the persons who <u>succeed</u> at losing a lot of weight eventually <u>fail</u> at keeping that weight off?*

The weight control world has spent years trying to discover the answer to that head-scratcher. But, as best I can see, all the research and theorizing has failed to identify the true cause.

So, what is the true reason why about ninety percent of the persons who succeed at losing a lot of weight eventually fail at keeping that weight off, while ten percent succeed at it?

Here, in my opinion, is why that happens.

In weight control studies, a hundred percent of the persons cited have already succeeded at weight reduction. They've succeeded at weight reduction because they've all applied the 3-step Process to Weight Success (although they may have not recognized it at the time).

That is, they made a decision to take their body weight down to a certain number (the decision step). They selected a specific weight-reduction action plan for accomplish-ing it (the action plan selection step). And, finally, they did the plan (the daily do-it step). *This resulted in them succeeding at their weight-reduction pursuit.*

Then, after succeeding at weight reduction a strange thing happened to the group. Ninety percent of the study participants went one direction and ten percent went another direction. That is, ninety percent *stopped* doing the daily do-it step (step 3) and ten percent *continued* doing the daily do-it step. Or, in other words, ninety percent went into "do-nothing mode" and ten percent went into "weight maintenance mode."

And, what was the outcome? The group in "do-nothing mode" gained back all the weight they lost. And, conversely, the group in "weight maintenance mode" maintained their desired weight for the rest of their life.

Or, put another way, what happened is this. For ninety percent of the persons, once they achieved their weight loss goal they ceased pursuing weight management. But, for ten percent of the persons, once they achieved their weight loss goal they adopted a *weight maintenance goal.* Then they commenced pursuing this goal with as much determination as they put into pursuing their weight loss goal. In other words, they never quit performing the daily do-it actions of Step 3. They just changed the target.

So, to sum up, the difference between the ninety percent who regained the lost weight and the ten percent who kept it off is this.

(1) The ninety percent who lost weight and then gained it back applied the 3-step Process to Weight Success during the weight reduction stage only, and

(2) the ten percent who kept the weight off applied the 3-step Process for both the weight reduction stage _and_ the weight maintenance stage. Or, in short, they kept doing Step 3 for the rest of their life.

Now here's what you need to know: _Anyone_ can be in the "ten percent group," provided that they do the 3-step Process to Weight Success for both the weight reduction stage _and_ the weight maintenance stage.

A popular myth is that weight maintenance is harder than weight reduction. People come to that conclusion because they've been applying the "do-nothing" approach for their "weight maintenance stage." But when persons apply the 3-step Process to Weight Success to their weight maintenance stage, I believe it turns out that weight maintenance is *easier* than weight reduction.

So, to say it again, the main difference between those who lose weight and then gain it back and those who lose weight and then keep it off is this:

Those who are keeping it off are continuing to do Step 3 for the rest of their life.

Or, put another way, they're continuing to do a set of daily weight-success-creating actions **every** day (or at least most days).

How to Succeed at Lifelong Weight Maintenance

So we now know that the big key to creating lifelong weight success is to do Step 3 — the Daily Do-it Step — for the rest of one's life. But for many persons, once they get into weight maintenance stage something goes awry. It happens like this.

After succeeding at weight reduction these persons enter their weight maintenance stage with vigor and commitment. They continue doing the actions prescribed in their eating action plan. And they get good results from it.

But then gradually a bad condition sneaks in. Over time, the person begins to drift away from doing the actions specified in their eating action plan. At first they fail to do it only a couple days a month. But then pretty soon they're failing to do it two or three days a week. And, eventually ... they're no longer doing it at all. In short, they self-sabotage their weight success journey without even realizing it. This condition is widespread and has been around for decades. I call it *weight maintenance self-sabotage.*

And what's the result of weight mainte-nance self-sabotage? The person gains back all the weight they worked so hard to lose a year or two earlier. This now brings us to a key question: How does a person avoid weight maintenance self-sabotage? Or, put another way, *how does a person stay focused on doing their chosen eating action plan for the rest of their life?*

The answer is: Create a Personal Daily Focus program. Then do it *every* day.

By doing a Personal Daily Focus program you cause your mind to point you toward doing the daily actions prescribed in your eating action plan for the rest of your life.

So, what actions might you include in your Personal Daily Focus program? Here are six suggested actions for you to consider. I call them *Mind-focusers.* You might do all of them, or only some of them — your choice.

> **Note:** In case you might like to know, these are the main actions in my own Personal Daily Focus program. I've been applying these actions since 2008 (and, as a result, have been living almost every day of that time in my desired healthy-weight range).

So, here for your consideration and possible use are six daily mind-focusers for succeeding at creating lifelong desired weight maintenance.

1 – Weight Range Goal
2 – Daily Weighing
3 – Daily Self-praise
4 – Goal Statement Iteration
5 – Weight Success Benefits Recitation
6 – Reminder System

> **Note:** You don't need to do all six to get good results. Even just one can have a powerful impact on causing you to do Step 3 for the rest of your life. But, of course, the more you do, the better.

MIND-FOCUSER #1: Weight Range Goal

Instead of having a single number as your weight goal, have a weight *range* — which we call Desired Weight Range. Make your desired weight range to be, say, eight to ten pounds (or four to five kilos). So each day that your weight is in your desired weight range, *you view yourself as being a **Weight Winner.*** To illustrate, if your desired weight range is, say, 155–165 pounds, then every day that your weight is between 155.0 to 165.9 pounds you are a Weight Winner. And you should feel great about it.

> **Note:** Your desired weight range isn't fixed for life. Whenever conditions call for it, you can adjust your desired weight range to a more appropriate one.

MIND-FOCUSER #2: Daily Weighing

Forget about weekly weighing. Instead, do accurate DAILY weighing. For optimal results, apply these eight rules.

1 – Use a good scale — one that's consistently accurate. Use the *same* scale for each weighing.

2 – Weigh at the *same* time, or in the *same* hour, each day (and weigh only once a day). My personal experience is that the best time is prior to breakfast.

3 – Avoid eating before weighing.

4 – Empty your bladder before weighing.

5 – Weigh yourself with nothing on, or else with the *same* weight of clothing each time.

6 – Position the scale on the *same* spot on the floor.

7 – Stand on the *same* spot on the scale.

8 – Use the *same* weight distribution on your feet. It doesn't matter what the weight distribution is as long as it's the same with each weighing.

THEN, once the weight number comes up on the scale, *SAY* that number to yourself (preferably aloud if the situation allows). Do this <u>every</u> day.

MIND-FOCUSER #3: Daily Self-praise

If you're doing your chosen eating action plan every day (that is, you're doing Step 3 of the 3-step Process), then your daily weighing number will be in your desired weight range on most days. Every time that happens do this. Deliver appreciation and praise to your mind. Do it with exuberance and joy. Here's some sample wording for it.

"My dear Mind — thank you, thank you, thank you for guiding me to living yet another day in my desired weight range. I truly appreciate you doing it. Please keep it

up. Keep on creating daily thoughts and feelings that guide me to consuming the **types** of food and the **amount** of food that results in me living each day of the rest of my life in my desired healthy-weight range."

MIND-FOCUSER #4: Goal Statement Iteration

Create a healthy-weight goal statement, and then say it to yourself at least **25** times each day. To make it easy for you, here's a tidy, easy-to-remember statement:

> I <u>am</u> the person of my healthy weight.
> I am healthy, happy, and doing great.

> **Note:** For our purpose here, we assume every weight in your desired weight range (see Mind-focuser #1) is a healthy weight for you.

Does saying it 25 times a day seem like it would be time-consuming? It's not. You're probably able to say your Goal Statement *three times* in 12 to 15 seconds, which is 12 to 15 times a minute. Which means, saying it 25 times per day uses *less than* 120 seconds per day.

Plus, the Goal Statement need not be said all at once. You can divide it into several sessions. Or, if you like, you can spread it throughout the day.

Plus, you can say it aloud, either in full voice or in a whisper. Or, you can say it silently to yourself — your choice. So, you can do it *any time, any place.*

Plus, here's an easy way to keep track of your goal statement iterations: Count them in units of five using one of your hands. After each iteration move one of your fingers (either in or out). After moving all five fingers, say the total number to that point. So, after counting the first five say "Five" (either aloud or silently), after the second five say "Ten," after the third five "Fifteen," and so on.

Even though you can say your Goal Statement any time you want, some particularly
good times to say it are (a) when you
awaken in the morning, (b) whenever you
feel an urge to eat, (c) while you're eating,
(d) before you go to sleep at night, and (e)
whenever you wake up in the night. Saying
it at these times can have extra-powerful
impact.

MIND-FOCUSER #5: Weight Success Benefits Recitation

Succeeding at lifelong weight maintenance
often requires more than just focusing on a
weight goal. It helps greatly to also stay
aware of the *benefits* derived from that goal.

So, I suggest you create a list of all the
good things that will come your way from
living in your healthy-weight range. We call
these good things *weight success benefits.*
To make your benefits listing job easy I've

provided a list of twenty possible benefits. Of course, *you should ignore those that don't apply to you.* Plus you should add in any benefit that does apply but isn't on the list. Your final list can include both general benefits and specific. Use whatever wording carries the most meaning for you.

List of Possible Weight Success Benefits

1. I have a greater chance of *living healthier longer* — or greater chance of living free of debilitating accidents, illnesses, and bodily malfunction.

2. I experience greater happiness, including a daily good feeling from succeeding at creating lifelong healthy-weight living.

3. I experience greater eating pleasure.

4. I feel better.

5. I look better.

6. I move better.

7. I have greater agility.

8. I have greater energy and stamina.

9. I have enhanced self-image and self-esteem.

10. I have better overall health and fewer annoying ailments.

11. My clothes fit better and feel more comfortable.

12. I'm no longer constantly growing out of clothes.

13. I can do more [of a particular fun thing or things].

14. I eliminate [a particular illness or affliction].

15. I improve [a particular relationship].

16. I overcome [a particular problem].

17. I can better engage in [a particular activity or pursuit].

18. I have a greater chance of avoiding debilitating physical accidents, such as falling down.

19. I have a greater chance of living longer.

20. I will be more active in my latter years.

Then, once you've created your *My Weight Success Benefits* list, **read it every day.**

MIND-FOCUSER #6: Reminder System

One of the biggest causes of weight control failure is failure to *remember* to do what one should be doing. In other words, we can have a good eating action plan and have a desire to perform it <u>but</u> in the hustle-bustle of daily life we often forget to do it.

So, set up a reminder mechanism that will remind you each day to perform the actions prescribed by your eating action plan (that you selected during Step 2).

For example, make reminder messages to yourself. Then place these messages where you'll see them every day. Possibilities include: (a) in your bedroom, (b) on the refrigerator, (c) in your wallet or purse, (d) in your car, (e) on your computer, and (f) on your exercise equipment. Plus, put digital messages on your computer screen, smartphone, and other devices. In short, do whatever it takes to create a *failproof* reminder system.

> **Note:** If it happens you'd like to check out some additional Mind-focusers get the book titled *The Key to Weight Success* and then read Chapter **18: Six More Mind Motivators.**

THE ULTIMATE SOLUTION TO AN UNACCEPTABLE SITUATION

If you've been diligently applying a particular dietary or weight success action plan — that is, you've been doing every action the plan calls for you to do — and the results you've been getting are unacceptable, what should you do? (Note: "Unacceptable results" would be when you're in weight reduction stage and you haven't been losing weight or when you're in weight maintenance stage and you've been gaining weight.)

Simply put, when you're diligently applying a particular eating (or dietary) action plan and you've been getting ongoing unacceptable results, you should *replace* your present action plan with a new one — one that you believe will be more effective for you.

Now here's three concepts you should keep in mind.

(1) If you're doing every action called for by your eating action plan <u>and</u> you're not getting acceptable results, that means you have the *wrong* action plan for you.

(2) If you have the *right* action plan for you <u>and</u> you do everything called for by the plan, you *will* get acceptable results.

(3) If you don't presently have the optimal action plan for you, that doesn't mean such a plan doesn't exist. Somewhere in the weight management world there <u>is</u> an eating action plan, or dietary program, that will work for *you.*

∗　　∗　　∗

To conclude, I wish you the best on your lifelong weight success journey. I'm confident you'll end up living most or all of the rest of your days in your desired healthy-weight range <u>and</u> derive many well-deserved benefits from it.

> **Optional Additional Tools:** If it happens you'd like to check out even more tools for expediting your weight success journey, go to: correllconcepts.com/toolkit.pdf　(It's free.)